The Biochem

A handy guide for prescri...
Dr. Schuessler's Biochemic Tissue Salts

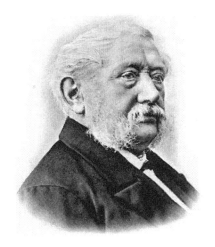

By **Prashant S. Shah**

Available from Amazon and Kindle online bookstore

ISBN-13: 978-1535061735
ISBN-10: 1535061731
ASIN: B01FA6X4FG

Address: H-901 Nilamber Bellissimo, Vasna-Bhayli Road, Vadodara 391 410, Gujarat, India.
Email: prashantshah@alum.mit.edu
Site on Internet at http://spiritual-living.in

A Disclaimer

The ideas on healing and the biochemic remedies suggested in this book are given for self-help. It is up to you, the reader, to make a proper and effective use of them. The author and publisher of this book do not accept any liability that may arise directly or indirectly from using this book.

Contents

SOME REVIEWS

Dr. S. V. Dixit (Homeopath)

This book has what you really need to make a prescription; and what is more important is that it doesn't have what you don't need! It is not superfluous or overloaded with symptoms. So, it is a real time saver... The writing is clear and to the point. The small size of the book should make it a favourite of housewives, for whom I take it that this book is really intended. I strongly recommend this book.

Nicole C. Nurse

This (Biochemic) therapy is very popular in Germany. Every second household uses these cell salts... I've read many books on Biochemic cell-salts, but this book is more up-to-date and very clear! Plus it tells how the healing happens inside the living body. I found it very useful and insightful. The author should write more.

Saket S. Vaidya, Consulting Engineer

These Biochemic remedies are surprisingly very effective. You can feel the effect after taking just a few doses. The write-up (book) is compact, and yet in a few pages it gives us a wide understanding (encyclopaedic) of how the human body functions. The more I read these pages, the more insight I get on how the human body is designed to function; what causes imbalance in our body; and how these vibrated tissue salts (remedies) actually go about restoring our health. I've studied this manuscript and it has really helped me understand my constitution. Now I feel better equipped and more confident about solving my health problems. This book and a box of 12 tissue remedies are some of the best investments I have made.

Sanjeev Vaidya, Retired Engineer

The biochemic remedies are truly effective. Some time back my wife had an acidity problem. I was able to help her with Nat Phos. It gave quick relief and now the frequency of the trouble has reduced considerably. In another case, there were painful knots in the breast. They completely disappeared after treatment with just a few doses of Calc Flour... The uniqueness of the book is that it is handy (small) and without confusion. It should prove to be a great help to the common person for maintaining health in the family.

Marsha Carter, On Amazon

Well thought out and very well written (book)! This is not a superficial book – it is concise and simple and not a detailed text book. Each salt is well explained, but briefly; and salts are contrasted to give a better understanding of each. I highly recommend this book to those who want to actually use the cell salts.

Ms. B, On Amazon

A small book full of great information on cell salts. These cell salts are not dangerous to use, so anyone can use them to benefit their family and friends. The generalized aspects of healing are very well explained in this wonderful book. However, I also need one that describes more deeply the 'bullet points' that are offered here. Definitely one (book) for your library; highly recommended if you are only going to use just one book on cell salts.

AUTHOR'S PREFACE

Allopathic medicine is the mainstream system. It is a leader for treatment in emergencies, in infectious diseases, and for ailments that require surgical intervention. However, most of the common troubles that we face are only FUNCTIONAL DISORDERS, like:

respiratory disorders – the common cold and cough;

skin disorders – rashes that itch, dandruff and foul odour;

pains – headache, stiff-joints and back pains; and

digestive disorders – irritable bowels, constipation and flatulence.

And for such disorders the allopathic (modern) medical system has no effective remedy! The doctor only tries to manage or relieve the annoying symptoms of a disorder so as to provide some temporary relief; and during this time the body tries to heal itself. However, when you give this kind of treatment, the acute symptoms of the disorder get modified into chronic disorders such as headaches, stuffy nose, acidity, gas trouble, rheumatic pain, skin rashes, respiratory allergy (like asthma, wheezing), high blood pressure, etc. These newer symptoms are less intense in their effects, but they *harass more* since they last for a long time and recur periodically. Very often the patient has to be put on some medication, which has to be continued for a lifetime!

A striking contrast to this modern approach to healing is found in the classical system of Biochemic Remedies. When you treat a disorder with tissue salts, you don't suppress the symptoms. Hence, the acute symptoms don't get converted into chronic disorders. You *merely use the symptoms to diagnose* the appropriate biochemic remedy that is necessary in each case. The remedy will stimulate the body's vital force and make it more responsive. Then vital force takes over and eliminates the toxins from the body tissues. When the toxin level is sufficiently reduced, the natural functions of the body get restored and the body returns to health.

The biochemic system is 'HOLISTIC' since it relies on restoring the body's vital force. The vital force is an 'overall principle', which is not confined to any part of the body. And this force is restored by administering the appropriate tissue salt *as a vibration* (potency) that is generated in sugar of milk. Thus, the healing happens through a natural process.

NOTE: In the Biochemical system the vital force is a power in our 'energy body'. This power animates our physical body and keeps it working as a whole. It is only when the vital force becomes insufficient that the individual body parts of the body become susceptible to disorders and infections.

This Biochemic system is simple to understand and easy to use. And further, it comes without the 'side-effects' that normally arise from using the drug therapy. Still further, you have to select a remedy from just 12 tissue salts. And to make the selection you don't need to know the nature of a disease in detail or depend on expensive laboratory test and investigation. My mother used to treat us (family) with these biochemic remedies when we were kids. And she did a pretty good job with it even though she had no training in healthcare!

To be able to treat the patient or yourself effectively, you have to only study the 'guiding symptoms' indicated for each of the 12 Biochemic remedies. I have personally used these Biochemic remedies, and over the years I have found the results to be consistent and very satisfactory.

This book is *written from experience*. Great care is taken to characterise the signature of each tissue-salt. You have to only read the short description of the tissue-salts to be able to diagnose the remedy. And in finding this remedy you don't have to search through a large number of symptoms and remedies, as in Homeopathy.

With a little practice in the art of prescribing, you can *become a domestic physician* (not a licensed physician). Then you can safely help yourself, your family and your friends in health matters. It will overcome your helplessness on health issues and reduce your unnecessary dependence on the medical profession.

The *new second edition* of the book has many improvements: The chapter **'Tips for Differentiating the Remedies'** is added; and the chapter on **'Remedies for Classified Diseases'** is totally revised. These improvements will make it much easier for you to diagnose the correct Biochemic remedy in each case and to use it more effectively.

Prashant S. Shah

* Most common troubles that we are faced with are functional disorders, and for such troubles the allopathic (modern) medical system has no effective remedy!

* To be able to treat the patient or yourself effectively, you have to only study the 'guiding symptoms' indicated for each of the twelve Biochemic remedies.

A SYNOPSIS

Biochemic medicine was discovered over a hundred years ago by a German physician, Dr. Wilhelm Heinrich Schuessler. He analysed the ash content of human cells and identified twelve inorganic tissue-salts that are essential for the healthy functioning of the human body.

He showed that when there is a deficiency of any of these salts in the body tissues, certain typical symptoms arise. You can use these symptoms *to identify* the specific deficiency in the patient.

Then all you have to do is supplement the deficient tissue-salt in a dynamic form (6X potency). It will stimulate the vital force of the body, which will in turn carry out the healing.

Here is an up-to-date, clear, and concise book. You can use it to heal yourself, your family and friends. It tells you how the common everyday ailments arise in the body and how to use the tissue salts to heal them. The book is simple to understand and easy to use; and the results are simply amazing.

INTRODUCTION

In the 18th century there was great interest in the biochemistry of cells. In 1873, Dr. Schuessler analysed the ash content of human cells and identified twelve inorganic tissue salts that are essential for the healthy functioning of the human body.

He believed that there is a *biochemical basis* to cellular health and vitality of the body organs, and they are maintained by a balance of these twelve tissue salts. Thus, these inorganic tissue-salts were considered to play a vital role in healthy functioning of the human body: in digesting food; in assimilating nutrients; and in eliminating the biological waste products.

Whenever there is a deficiency of any of these inorganic salts in the body tissues, certain typical symptoms are found to arise in the patient. So, when you observe such symptoms in a person, all you have to do is supply the deficient tissue-salt in a potentised form (6X). It will stimulate the vital force of the body, which will do the healing.

Dr. Schuessler administered these tissue-salts in a

potentised or vibrated form. More often he used the 6X potency.

In this therapy you do not suppress the symptoms of a disease to give immediate relief and claim a cure. Instead you focus on restoring the healing power of the vital force and allow it to do the healing through a natural process. Further, you consider the healing to happen through a biochemical process. For this reason these 'inorganic salt supplements' are called 'Biochemic Remedies' or simply *Biochemic tissue-salts*. They can be purchased in the potentialised form (6X) from most Homeopathic Pharmacies and online stores.

The twelve Biochemic tissue salts are as follows:

1) Calcarea fluor (Calcium fluoride)
2) Calcarea phos (Calcium phosphate)
3) Calcarea sulf (Plaster of Paris - Calcium sulphate)
4) Ferrum phos (Iron phosphate)
5) Kali mur (Potassium chloride)
6) Kali phos (Potassium phosphate)
7) Kali sulf (Potassium sulphate)
8) Magnesia phos (Magnesium phosphate)
9) Natrum mur (Sodium chloride)

10) Natrum phos (Sodium phosphate)
11) Natrum sulf (Glauber's salt - Sodium sulphate)
12) Silicea (Silica).

These inorganic salts are present in the blood, lymph, bone, nerves, etc. Whenever there is a *deficiency* of one or more of these tissue-salts in the body organs, certain typical symptoms arise in the body. The biochemic *remedy* in all such cases is to stimulate the vital force of the body with a potentised form of the deficient tissue salt. Then the vital force will be restored, and the body will on its own overcome its deficiency and begin to heal itself.

It is interesting to note that Dr. Schuessler was originally a Homoeopath. Hence, over the years this Biochemic system has been given a *supportive role* in Homeopathic treatment. However, the basis for selecting the remedy in these two systems is different. In Biochemic system you are supplementing a *'deficiency'* of the tissue-salts; whereas in the Homoeopathic system you use the remedy according to the *'law of cure'* (let likes be treated by likes). The main thing in common is that the remedies are administered in a *'potentised form'*. That is, they are given as pills of sugar of milk, which contains a vibration of the inorganic salt. There is no active chemical substance as in the drug therapy.

This Biochemic system is much simpler than its parent, Homoeopathy. Here you choose the remedy from the guiding symptoms of just twelve tissue-salts! On the other hand, in Homoeopathy you have to collect a very wide range of symptoms, repertories them, and then find the matching remedy from an equally large number of remedies. Hence, the task can be overwhelming.

Many books on Biochemic Remedies are available in the market. However, most of them have been written in the 'old style' – as a collection of symptoms. As a result these books carry the complexity of the 'homoeopathic drug-picture'. It has made this very simple Biochemic system unnecessarily complicated and confusing.

In this book we have clarified this confusion. We have made simple descriptions of the 'guiding symptoms' for each Biochemic remedy. You have to only grasp them to make your prescription.

In addition, here we also explain the process of

healing in the body — how the vital force goes about overcoming the symptoms of the illness. It is always helpful to know what to expect when you are waiting for the healing to happen inside the body.

Dr. Schuessler analysed the ash content of human cells and identified twelve inorganic tissue salts that are essential for the healthy functioning of the body.

Whenever certain symptoms arise in the body, they are considered to arise from a deficiency of one or more of these tissue-salts.

The biochemic remedy in all such cases is to stimulate the vital force of the body with a potentised form of the deficient tissue salt.

Then the vital force will be restored, and the body will on its own overcome its deficiency and begin to heal itself.

THE GUIDING SYMPTOMS

In this Biochemic system the tissue-salts are prescribed on the basis of the guiding symptoms that prevail in the patient. The remedies are not selected according to the classification of diseases.

These biochemic tissue salts are useful in treating functional disorders, and also many chronic or constitutional health disorders. Hence, in addition to the guiding symptoms we have also indicated the kinds of ailments or therapeutic conditions that can be treated with these tissue salts. The discussion is conceptual. Great care is taken to bring out the characteristic effects or the signature of each tissue-salt. The description will help you in recognising the indicated remedy in each case.

The salts are listed in following order:

- Calcium salts
- Iron (Ferrum) salt
- Potassium (Kali) salts
- Magnesium salt
- Sodium (Natrum) salts
- Silicea

Calcarea Fluor

This salt is the main constituent of tooth enamel and the *elastic fibre* of all muscular and connective tissues. Hence, you can use it when the skin, muscles, ligaments and/or the blood vessels have lost their elasticity, are sagging, or have become lax. It tones up the smooth muscles that have lost their flexibility and elasticity (chronic dilation).

Thus, Cal flour will heal a prolapsed uterus; a bladder or uterus with a dragging down sensation; haemorrhoids that have enlarged; joints that dislocate easily; glands that have hardened or calcified (since the exudation of waste was difficult); skin that is cracked or sagging; and veins that have become varicose (swollen and prominent).

It will tighten the gums around the teeth and prevent them from receding. It will soften the lumps that develop on bones (after a bad bruise to a bone or a fracture) or around joints (after a bad sprain). It will strengthen the *bones* that are bending (as in bow legs or hunched back); and break down the spurs that develop osteoarthritis.

In respiratory ailments the deficiency of this tissue

salt causes the discharges from the nose, throat or chest to be typically thick, yellow and lumpy.

Cal flour is a great remedy for *stiffness* in cartilages: It will relieve backaches and joint pains that become worse on beginning to move and get better with continued movement. Its action is similar to the remedy *Rhus Tox* in homeopathy. It also has similarities with *Ruta* and *Calcarea Carb*. The symptoms are usually worse in wet weather.

The clinical conditions for Cal Fluor:

- Weak enamel of teeth
- Fissure (cracks) in gums
- Receded gums
- Prolapsed uterus
- Varicose veins
- Uterus displacements
- Hernia
- Fistula
- Piles
- Internal haemorrhoids
- Anal fissures
- Spurs in joints (osteoarthritis)

- Cataract (in eye)
- Rough and cracked skin (of hands)
- Knotty lymphatic glands
- Calcification of glands
- Sagging of facial tissues
- Weakness in tendons and ligaments
- Cysts (membranous sac containing fluid)
- Fibroids (a benign tumour)
- Hard warts

Guiding symptoms for Cal Flour

Indicated mainly in	Loss of **elasticity**: dilated, relaxed or sagging of muscle tissue. Cracks in skin. Worn out enamel in teeth. Hardening of glands. Stiffness in body. Sluggish circulation; Skeletal weakness (like bow legs). *Mental*: Fear of financial ruin; pessimistic.
Tongue	Dry, cracked, swollen.
Discharges	Nose: Thick, lumpy greenish yellow discharge. Expectoration: Tiny lumps of tough yellow mucus with offensive smell. Ulcers: Having thick yellow pus.
> Worse by	> Wet weather, after rest, and on beginning to move.
< Better by	< By rubbing, hot applications, and continued movement.

Calcarea Phos

This salt is associated with *defective nutrition* in bones, muscles, and glands; and with teething troubles in children.

Cal phos is an essential mineral in gastric juices that are necessary for assimilating proteins. Hence, it is given for *building* the blood cells (anaemia), muscles (strength) and bones (as in teething).

It is commonly used as a tonic to quicken recovery after an illness or after exhausting albuminous discharges and menopause. It will relieve vertigo due to weakness. This remedy is similar to the homeopathic *China and Chamomile.*

The indications for this salt are foul taste in the mouth, bloating in the stomach, or heartburn. Often the person cannot bear tight clothing.

A deficiency of this salt gives rise to *aching pains* in bones, joints and muscles. Often the lower limbs become weak or numb. Use it to heal brittle bones or cracked bones, as in a fracture.

It is most commonly used for a quick recovery after an acute illness; after wasting diseases like TB; for effects of sexual excess; and for emotional disorders.

Usually the patient is very sensitive to the cold and drafts. He or she has a tendency to catch a cold or develop a stiff neck.

This remedy is very useful for school girls that are undergoing hormone imbalance. There is restless; swaying of emotions; and freckles or pimples on the face.

Many symptoms of Cal Phos arise after every change of weather.

The clinical conditions for Cal Phos:

- Weak or brittle bones
- Abnormal bone growth
- Rickets (Vitamin D deficiency)
- Difficulty in teething
- Dental caries (tooth decay)
- Lumbago
- Aching in bones, joints & muscles
- Digestive disorders due to poor assimilation
- Bloated tummy
- Chronic enlargement of tonsils (colds settle here)

- Pimples, acne, eczema
- Worms

Guiding symptoms for Cal Phos

Indicated mainly in	Weak **nutrition**: Poor assimilation of calcium and protein. Deficiency in bones; teething troubles. Weakness in general. Stiffness and aching in muscles, joints cartilages and bones. *Mental*: Effect of jealousy; restless; emotionally fragile.
State of tongue	Stiff, numb; dry; blister on tip; bad or bitter taste in morning.
Discharges	Nose & throat: **albuminous** (thick clear like the white of raw egg). Skin: Itching with pimples and eruptions. Digestive tract: Belching; bloated.
> Worse by	> Getting wet, cold, motion, jealousy, **changes in weather**.
< Better by	< Warmth and rest

Calcarea Sulf

The main function of this cell-salt is to remove impurities (like pus) from blood. These impurities show their effect on the mucous membranes and the skin.

Thus, it will finish boils or abscesses that are discharging, but not healing; it will close the wounds have become infected and are filled with thick yellow pus, which are lumpy or blood-streaked; it will also cleanse fungal infections. The cleansing action of this salt is similar to the homeopathic *Hepar sulph*.

The different organs of the body cannot perform their tasks well when the blood becomes toxic with pus. Hence, this salt is often used as an inter-current remedy while treating *chronic* conditions like coughs, colds, earaches, eczemas, and eye infections. Use it when the indicated remedy does not work.

The discharges are characteristically thick and yellow. It also serves as an expectorant in chest congestions. It opens up the congested mucus plugs.

The clinical conditions for Cal Sulf:

- Suppurating wounds
- Skin and ear abscess
- Conjunctivitis with thick yellow discharge
- Furuncles (single big boil)
- Carbuncles (many headed boil)
- Gumboil
- Fungal skin infections
- Chronic eczema with scabs
- Leucorrhea (a thick, whitish or yellowish vaginal discharge)
- Herpes (second stage)
- Bronchitis (third stage)
- Chronic Acne
- Cystic Tumors

Guiding symptoms for Cal Sulf

Indicated mainly in	**Anti-septic** and blood purifier: Use after suppuration to make the inflamed part discharge its accumulated pus and avoid slow decay; useful in chronic catarrhs, carbuncles, abscesses and ulcers that don't heal easily. *Mental*: Discontented, sad, lazy.
State of tongue	Flabby; clay coloured, sour, soapy or acrid taste in the mouth. Inflamed with sores.
Discharges	Thick, yellow and purulent, sometimes mixed with blood. Skin: Forms scabs (crust over wounds); dry eczema.
> Worse by	> Getting wet.
< Better by	< Warmth and dry open air.

Ferrum Phos

This salt is a constituent of the red blood corpuscles, which act as the carrier of oxygen to the different parts of the body. Use it whenever there is an indication of infection or inflammation in any part of the body (heat, redness and pain).

Usually the temperature rises to fight the bacteria or virus, and unless it rises beyond 102 degrees F, it should not be suppressed with drugs or cold applications. This cell-salt is most useful at this stage. It is the Biochemic 'rescue remedy' for the first stage in all acute illnesses.

Thus, *Ferrum phos* is used in the first stage of fevers; and at the onset of an acute respiratory illnesses (like coughs or colds), *before* any swellings or discharges have developed. The patient will be listless, there will be redness of parts, but other symptoms may not have developed. Its action is similar to the homeopathic *Belladonna*.

This salt is useful when the muscle fibres are relaxed. Often there is *dilation* with an accumulation of blood, and sometimes there is also some haemorrhage. It is the first remedy for earaches or nosebleeds after an injury.

Use it in simple cases of anaemia or lowered vitality. You can alternate it with *Calc phos.* The 'calcium' will help the body to absorb the iron more effectively. *Ferrum phos* is an excellent iron tonic and it does not have the 'side effects' that arise from using the usual iron supplements.

The clinical conditions for Ferrum Phos:

- Rescue remedy in infections, inflammations and fevers
- Anemia
- Vertigo
- headache
- Hemorrhages (bleeding)
- Bleeding hemorrhoids
- Colitis (first stage of infection of colon)
- Recurrent colds and hay fever (builds immunity)
- Tonsillitis, Laryngitis, Bronchitis Conjunctivitis, Mastitis
- Earache
- Croup (inflammation of larynx or trachea)

- Acute rheumatism
- Low blood pressure

The guiding symptoms for Ferrum Phos

Indicated mainly in	**Anti-inflammatory**: Use in first stage of inflammations, fevers, pains and colds (respiratory tract) – before the onset of pus or mucus discharges. *Mental*: Listless; dull; Loss of courage or hope.
State of tongue	Clean & red; throat is dry and inflamed (red).
Discharges	Dryness of mucus membrane, burning sensation. Expectoration: Scanty, streaked with blood. Haemorrhage: Bright red blood, which coagulates easily.
> Worse by	> Heat, motion.
< Better by	< Cold applications, after rest.

Kali Mur

This cell salt unites with albumen (protein) to form fibrin, which is found in all tissues of the body except bone. When *Kali mur* is deficient, the fibrin becomes non-functional and gives rise to a thick, whitish discharge from the mucus membranes. It gives rise to a typical *white coating* on the tongue.

Kali mur is most useful in treating the second stage of inflammations and congestions. It is helpful in all catarrhal conditions such as coughs, stuffy head colds, chest colds or stuffed sinuses, etc. where there is swelling or white discharge. There may be white ulcers or thrush in the mouth. It is similar to homeopathic *Phytolacta, Mercurious* and *Bryonia*.

This salt will relieve rheumatic swellings and detoxify the lymph and glandular systems of the body. It is very useful in treating earaches where there is congestion in the Eustachian tubes (so that hearing is affected). It will relieve the crackle and popping noises in the ears that arise after a cold.

The skin is dry with white scales. The eczema is also dry. This salt is the biochemic 'first aid' for burns and blisters. It heals them faster.

Here the digestion is always sluggish and the bile is lacking. There is indigestion or diarrhoea after consuming rich or fatty food.

The clinical conditions for Kali Mur:

- Sore throat
- Swollen gland
- Otitis; Tonsillitis; Pharyngitis; Bronchitis
- Diphtheria
- Thrush (sore mouth), canker in mouth
- Sluggish liver
- Indigestion after eating fatty food
- Colds, coughs and catarrh
- Herpes simplex (vesicles on outer surface of genitals)
- Measles
- Crusty eczema
- Soft warts
- Gastric catarrh
- Epilepsy from suppressed eruptions
- Bad effects after vaccination

Guiding symptoms for Kali Mur

Indicated mainly in	**Decongestant**: Sluggish constitution. Its deficiency makes fibrin non-functional; and it congests the mucus membranes of ear and throat. Use in the second stage of inflammation in catarrh, cough, boils, blisters and soft swellings (glands). *Mental*: Obstinate.
Tongue	Thick, **white or grey coating**.
Discharges	Thick, white, or slimy, mixed with phlegm. Stools: clay (light) coloured, deficient in bile; sometimes bloody. Skin: Eczema (dry, white crusts, with flour-like scales) and warts.
> Worse by	> **Eating rich or fatty food**; motion; night.
< Better by	< Rubbing; scratching; hot applications.

Kali Phos

It is the mineral constituent of the grey matter of nerve fibres, as in the brain. It is used as a 'nerve tonic' for people in the convalescent stage of any acute illness (especially after flu) where there is nervous exhaustion. Give it freely to people who are under the pressure of mental work or study (exams) or to executives who are experiencing a 'burn out'. The patient usually has a strong need for warmth and rest.

This salt relieves nervousness that arises from emotional stress. Hence, it is ideally suited to persons who *"fly of the handle for no good reason"*; or where there is hysteria, depression or tantrums.

The headache of *Kali phos* is often one-sided. There is great sensitivity to light and noise as in *Nux Vomica*), and the person is easily startled.

This salt is very useful in septic conditions where there is a *decay of the nerve* fibres. The fever is high (as in intestinal fever); the breath and body odour are foul (as in tooth decay); and the discharges are foul smelling and bloody (as in gangrene). The tongue has a mustard colour coating.

This salt is mostly used as a brain tonic to relieve nervousness, brain fag, insomnia (sleeplessness), and the condition of shattered nerves. It also relieves dull neuralgic pains. Its action is similar to the homeopathic *Phosphorus and Ignatia.*

The clinical conditions for Kali Phos:

- Ill-tempered children
- Tantrum
- Hysteria
- Phobias
- Insanity
- Mental illusions
- Hypochondriac (continuously worrying about health)
- Bed wetting
- Abnormal mental and physical weakness or lack of nerve energy.
- Nervousness without apparent cause
- Nervous headache, diarrhea, asthma, anxiety
- Neuralgic pains with fatigue
- Nerve degeneration

- Brain fag
- Stress related disorders
- Insomnia (sleepless)
- Pain in Shingles and Herpes
- Paralysis, Bells Palsy,
- Enuresis (involuntary urination)
- Vertigo
- Dysentery
- Typhoid
- Malignant troubles, Gangrene
- Menses: premature, profuse or offensive

Guiding symptoms for Kali Phos

Indicated mainly in	Nerve (grey matter) decay: Wasting diseases; degeneration of nerves and muscles; neuralgic pains; brain fag; insomnia; nervous headache; high fevers, intestinal fevers. *Mental*: Nervous, moody, tantrums, hysteria, indignation.

State of tongue	Brownish, like mustard; very dry and swollen in morning; foul taste; bad breath.
Discharges	Profuse, creamy yellow; thin and mixed with blood. Decay: Gangrene; very foul smelling. Eruptions: Burn, itch with greasy scabs. Blood in stools and vomit.
> Worse by	> Noise, **worry**, **excitement**, cold.
< Better by	< **Cheerful company**, eating, gentle motion.

Kali Sulf

This salt cleanses the skin, which is the largest organ of the body. Whereas *Ferrum phos* is the carrier of oxygen to the organs, *Kali sulf* is the transferor of oxygen onto the cells, where it is used. Hence, this tissue salt promotes 'cellular breathing'.

In this way it cleanses the epidermis (top layer of skin). It overcomes the dull and sickly appearance of the skin and scaling as in dandruff. It relieves psoriasis; and skin eruptions wherein the discharges are sticky and yellow, as in chicken pox.

The discharges from the mucus membranes are typically thick, sticky and yellow. The tongue is coated yellow.

When the skin discharges are suppressed, there is wheezing as in bronchitis (which is often worse between 3 to 5 AM).

Use this tissue salt in the 'third stage' of coughs, colds, earaches, etc. where some expectoration has formed. The expectoration is usually sticky and difficult to bring out.

Use it in inflammatory fevers to open up the pores of the skin and cause perspiration and internal (cellular) breathing. It relieves ailments that happen due to suppressed eruptions. The eruption usually returns in a milder form, and then passes away.

The remedy has many similarities with the homoeopathic *Pulsatilla* (**worse from heat and better in open air**). This remedy is indicated when there is change of weather from cold to warm. It brings out symptoms of a cough, cold, or rheumatic pains that typically move (shift) around in the body.

The clinical conditions for Kali Sulf:

- Psoriasis
- Eczema
- Ringworm
- Dandruff
- Ailments due to suppressed eruptions
- Measles
- Urticaria (a migrating rash with swelling), Nettlerash
- Seborrhea (oily skin secretion)
- Dermatitis (inflammation under the skin)
- Burning and itching eruptions
- Leucorrhea

- Bronchial asthma
- Chronic catarrhs
- Blocked nose
- Dropsy (swelling of soft tissues due to accumulation of water)
- Headaches
- Hormonal disturbances
- Lack of perspiration
- Tuberculosis
- Athlete's foot (fungal infection between the toes)
- Alopecia (sudden loss of hair; round patches in the scalp)

Guiding symptoms for Kali Sulf

Indicated mainly in	**Anti-inflammatory** – third stage in eruptive fevers to promote perspiration and internal breathing of the organ tissues. It relieves stuffy feeling, asthma, and allergic bronchitis. *Mental*: Timid & irritable; always hurrying.

State of tongue	Coated yellow, slimy, with whitish edges. Taste is lost with burning heat in mouth.
Discharges	Expectoration: Profuse and thin. Mucus membrane: Sticky, shiny, and yellowish-green discharge. Skin: Burning, dry, itching, profuse scaling or dandruff; ring worm; psoriasis; seasonal rashes.
> Worse by	> Evenings, warmth, & closed places.
< Better by	< Cool air, **open air**, motion.

Magnesia Phos

This salt has a striking effect on white-nerve fibres that spread out in the muscles. It is a general pain reliever in earache, headache, toothache (including teething in babies), abdominal colic, muscular spasms and even sciatica — as long as the pains are better by heat and pressure. For this reason it is called the 'biochemic aspirin'

The *characteristic* of the pain is sharp and spasmodic. It is like the cutting pains that come and go. It is not a dull pain! Here the muscles contract; so there is *convulsion, cramp and restlessness*. The action of this tissue salt is the opposite of Ferrum Phos, where there is relaxation.

The headaches have shooting pains and are better by warmth or wrapping (pressure).

This salt relieves painful menses, muscular twitching, hiccough and spasmodic coughs. Women who need this remedy may be found doubled up in bed with a hot water bottle pressed into their abdomen. It is best to take this cell-salt at the onset of the menses. The action of this tissue salt is similar to homeopathic *Colocynthis and Cimicifuga.*

Although this salt relieves the pains, it does not heal or remove the cause! However, it has no side effects. So it can be used it as often as necessary.

The effect of this salt is better when it is taken in warm water. Dissolve a few globules in half a glass of warm water and shake it vigorously with a plastic spoon. Then sip the water every few minutes to relieve the pain.

The clinical conditions for Mag Phos:

- Spasmodic asthma or cough
- Spasmodic menstrual cramps
- Spasm of the eyelid
- Nerve palpitation; Angina pectoris (heart)
- Convulsion
- Double vision
- Epileptic cramps
- Palsy (nerve disorder)
- Muscular cramps or twitching
- Colitis; abdominal colic
- Menstrual colic
- Sciatica

Guiding symptoms for Mag Phos

Indicated mainly in	**Anti-spasmodic** (white matter of nerves): Cramps; flatulent colic; abdominal or menstrual colic; darting or shooting pains; spasms; twitching. Hiccough; whooping cough. Cardiac (heart) pain. *Mental*: Keeps talking; impulsive; always complaining about pain.
State of tongue	Swollen and clean; or white coated in diarrhoea. Mouth: Dry with sticky saliva.
Discharges	Watery diarrhoea. Menstrual flow: Dark, clotted, intermittent.
> Worse by	> Open air, cold air, cold drinks, uncovering, motion, touching.
< Better by	< **Warmth**, hot drinks, applying **pressure, and bending over**

Natrum Mur

This salt affects the 'water balance' in mucous membranes, skin and body organs. There is *dryness* in the mouth along with strong thirst; lips are dry with a crack in the lower lip; the cough is dry and hacking; the bowels are dry and constipated etc. On the other hand the blood is thin and so the *discharges are watery*: the nose is running; the eyes are watering; there is much sneezing; or there is diarrhoea due to indigestion.

The unequal water distribution gives rise to circulation problems. Often the palms are sweaty and there is numbness in the limbs. There is oedema (excessive fluid build up in specific areas of the body) like puffy ankles; the creaking in joints (due to dryness). The mouth ulcers are dry and painful; and the blisters are water-filled like herpetic eruptions. And all these troubles are made worse by anxiety.

The patient has poor endurance to the heat of the Sun. It gives rise fluid imbalance in the brain. So, there is headache due to exposure to Sun. The headache is usually heavy, throbbing or hammering.

Food takes a long time to digest in the stomach. It gives rise to indigestion and a full sensation. As a result there is malnutrition even though the patient eats plenty.

Sometimes there is a salty taste in the mouth; excessive thirst; or craving for salt. And many troubles are aggravated near the seashore.

In catarrh *Nat mur* compares well with *Kali mur* and *Kali sulf*; in gastric troubles it compares well with *Nat sulf*; and in headache it compares well with *Cal phos* and *Ferr phos.*

Homoeopathy characterises the *Nat mur* person as being a *hypochondriac*: The person thinks too much about his or her ailment and feels hopeless. However, if you console them, they get irritated! The action of Biochemic *Nat mur* has many symptoms similar to Homeopathic *Sepia and Sulphur.*

The clinical conditions for Nat Mur:

- Watery discharges that burn and irritate
- Dry constipation or watery diarrhea
- Dry skin
- Chapped lips

- Colds with watery discharge
- Seaside asthma
- Excessive saliva
- Bronchitis with catarrh or watery mucus
- Watery vesicles
- Vaginal dryness
- Leucorrhea
- Pleurisy
- Profuse perspiration
- Dry cough
- Dry nose
- Snoring
- Sneezing, Hay fever
- Hives (nettle rash, Urticaria)
- Heavy or hammering headache
- Creaky joints
- Watery blisters; Herpes
- Oedema (water filled swellings)
- Thin watery blood
- Sun aggravations
- Insect bites (use as application)
- Hypochondriac (continuously worrying

about health)

Guiding symptoms for Nat Mur

Indicated mainly in	**Water distribution**: disproportionate – excessive moisture or dryness. Skin: Watery or dry; with eczema or herpetic eruptions. Oedema or dehydration. Intermittent fever like malaria (fever followed by sweating and chill); Heavy headache; Sun headache. Digestion is slow: Food stays undigested for too long; malnutrition. *Mental*: Irritable; defensive; depressed; feels helpless, but rejects consolation.
State of tongue	Dry, parched or covered with clear, frothy saliva; blisters on tip; salty taste. Throat: sore
Discharges	Secretions: Excessive; acrid;

	watery; salty; smarting, with sneezing; great thirst. (Or extreme dryness with itching, scales and crusts). Eruptions with watery content. Menses and leucorrhoea: Thin, watery.
> Worse by	>Mornings; grief; anger; anxiety; consolation; **seaside, periodic** complaints.
< Better by	< Evenings, cold, open air, pressure.

Natrum Phos

This salt maintains the *alkaline balance* in the body. It emulsifies fatty acids and keeps the uric acid soluble in the blood. It is helpful in troubles of the stomach and intestines when there is 'acidity' – a burning sensation with indigestion and gas. The digestive tract is very sensitive and *intolerant* to 'acid forming' foods like milk, fats, sweets, alcohol and vinegar. The person feels better by eating, but there is a sore feeling or sour belching 2 to 3 hours after eating.

There may be itching around the anus due to worms (which thrive in acidic conditions). There is constant picking of the nose or stitching pains in the liver region.

Sometimes constipation alternates with sour smelling and burning diarrhoea. Abdomen is bloated and there is involuntary flatulence.

The skin is sore, itching with rash; eczema with yellow scabs. Often there is eczema on the lower foot with intolerable itching.

All the discharges are characteristically sour smelling and creamy yellow.

This salt keeps urea soluble in the blood; otherwise uric acid salts can precipitate around joints and ligaments of the body and cause *stiffness* in skeletal muscles and *swellings* in joints. It relieves rheumatic conditions that arise due to acid diathesis; and it also serves as a kidney tonic. This remedy resembles the homoeopathic *Kali carb*, *Calc carb* and *Rheum*.

The clinical conditions for Nat Phos:

- Acidity of blood
- Acid reflux
- Sour belching; bloated abdomen
- Gastritis
- Dyspepsia
- Palpitation
- Gastric ulcer
- Colic due to acidity
- Gout
- Rheumatism (stiffness)
- Excessive, sour perspiration from feet and armpit
- Stitching pain in the liver or kidney
- Pain in joints
- Milk allergy

8,5

- Hives (nettle rash, Urticaria)
- Acne (pimples)
- Diabetes
- Diarrhea with burning
- Involuntary flatulence
- Frequent urination
- Worms
- Eyes glued together (morning)

Guiding symptoms for Nat Phos

Indicated mainly in	**Antacid**: Present in intercellular fluid and serves to split lactic acid into water & carbon dioxide. Malfunction: Acidity; deposits urea salts around joints – stiffness and swelling of joints. Headache: Frontal and temporal; worse in morning. Bloated abdomen; worms; diarrhoea; frequent urination; diabetes *Mental*: Anxious; forgetful; low self-esteem

State of tongue	Moist and creamy yellow coating at the back of tongue, like wash-leather. Acid taste. Hair like sensation
Discharges	From eyes, ears & skin: acidic, creamy yellow. Eructation: Sour, foul smelling. Skin: Eczema, itching, raw, with pimples or rash all over the body; yellow (honey coloured) scabs. Leucorrhoea: Acrid
> Worse by	> Thunder storm, noise, **open air**, sex, **before eating,** eating sweets, **milk**, sour food
< Better by	< Warmth, pressure, scratching, immediately after eating

Natrum Sulf

This salt is associated with the liver and it cleanses the intercellular fluids of the body.

Nat sulf is involved in carbohydrate metabolism in the body. Hence, it is useful in treating digestive upsets or nausea after eating starchy foods or fruits; and in morning diarrhoea where the stools are greenish.

It is called the 'liver salt' since the liver is often swollen, there is excessive bile (as in jaundice) and the gall bladder is sensitive. The taste is bitter, the tongue is coated dirty green-brown, and the discharges are greenish.

In some ways the action of this salt is the opposite of *Nat mur*: Both of them attract water, but in *Nat mur* the water is used by the organs to relieve their dryness, whereas in *Nat sulf* it is used to cleanse the cellular wastes from the cells and the intercellular fluid.

This salt is useful in treating intermittent fevers (that come and go); influenza with coughs and colds; rheumatism due to toxaemia; and headaches which are dull, frontal and occipital (at the base of the head). It also relieves the hangover that arises from taking excessive drinks.

A feeling of dullness and stuffiness in *damp or wet weather* always calls for this salt. This remedy has resemblance with the homoeopathic *Chelidonium, Bryonia* and *Thuja.*

The clinical conditions for Nat Sulf:

- Urine retention
- Bilious colic
- Vomiting of bitter bile
- All symptoms are aggravated by damp weather
- Stiffness, rheumatism
- Moist skin affections; wet eczema
- Jaundice
- Asthma in humid conditions
- Gonorrhea
- Bilious, fontal or occipital headache
- Malaria
- Flu (influenza)
- Tendency to form warts
- Flatulence, bloating

- Flushes of heat
- Enlarged prostate
- Oedema (swelling due to water retention) of feet

Guiding symptoms for Nat Sulf

Indicated mainly in	**Cleanser**: Cleans toxins from the intercellular fluids. Regulates carbohydrate metabolism. Relieves jaundice, rheumatism, humid asthma, flu, lethargy, and biliousness. Use in affections of the liver, kidney and gall bladder. *Mental*: Sad; must exercise restraint.
State of tongue	Dirty **greenish** brown coating. Mouth: Full of saliva; bitter taste.
Discharges	Nose: Pus changes to green on exposure to light. Cough: Green, thick, ropy. Diarrhoea: Bilious, green stools, with a lot of flatulence; reddish urine. Eruptions: *Moist* yellow scabs; warts.

> Worse by	> **Dampness,** wet weather, cold, mornings, breakfast.
< **Better** by	< Warm and dry weather; open air; passing flatus; and motion.

Silicea

The deficiency of this salt affects keratin, the fibrous tissue in the body. It gives rise to weakness in the *connective tissues* of bones, glands, hair, mucous membranes, nails, skin, teeth and nerves sheath. There is a typical brittleness of hair and nails; the skin develops wrinkles and cracks; jerks due to short circuit in nerves.

This salt will get rid of superfluous organic matter in the body. It functions like a *surgeon* in finishing abscesses, boils, carbuncles, corns and styes. It builds white blood cells; hastens suppuration or pus-formation process in boils and abscesses that are painful, but do not discharge easily. It extrudes foreign bodies like thorns from under the skin. In gout or rheumatic affections it pushes the tissues to throw out the accumulated waste. It acts on post-surgical scars that are inflamed, painful, and slow to heal.

It will relieve chronic swellings in glands, in the throat, in the ear, and of the sinuses.

This tissue-salt is most useful in *long continued infections* and in chronic skin disorders. The difference between the action of *Cal sulf* and *Sil* is that *Sil* ripens the abscess and promotes suppuration, whereas *Cal sulf* restrains the suppuration to cleanse and close the wound.

The *Silicea person* is typically sensitive, chilly, and sweaty; he catches cold easily; becomes chilled by cold wind; and lacks stamina and easily worn out by work. The body is imperfectly nourished due to deficient assimilation. The perspiration smells foul or it is suppressed; the skin itches; milk is not digested easily; there is nausea, and many symptoms are sensitive to the Moon phases, particularly to new and full Moon.

The clinical conditions for Silicea:

- Skin ulcers with tendency to suppurate
- Abscess
- Styes (boil on eyelid)
- Furuncles
- Carbuncles
- Tumors
- Tonsillitis with pus
- Suppuration of the bones
- Pustules

- Dermatitis
- Seborrhea (oily skin, inflammation of)
- Pneumonia
- Bronchitis
- Persistent ulcerations with fistula
- Herpes
- Scars after Measles
- Offensive perspiration
- Brittle or spotted nails
- In-growing nails
- Nail fungus
- Dry or cracking hair
- Ulcer of the cornea
- Anal fissures
- Corns in the foot
- Keloid scars (overgrowth of scar tissue around a wound)
- Prostate infections and enlargements
- Gonorrheal discharges
- White spotted nails
- Headaches in nape and forehead
- Alopecia (baldness)

- Chronic Asthma
- Troubles after vaccination
- Photophobia
- Gumboils
- Altitude sickness
- Weakness in the back
- Damaged ligaments

Guiding symptoms for Silicea

Indicated mainly in	**Surgeon's knife**: Promotes formation and extrusion of pus in inflamed parts of skin and connective tissues. Useful in ripening nasal catarrh, boils, gumboil, styes, tonsillitis, and liver abscess. It is slow and deep acting, and the gives lasting results. *Mental*: Over sensitive, shy, lacks confidence, and is easily discouraged.
State of tongue	Hardening of tongue, ulcers; sensation of hair.

Discharges	Skin: Pustules with yellow pus; weeping eczema; itching; offensive perspiration. Nails: Brittle, spotted. Face: Eruptions. Feet & armpit: offensive sweat. Expectoration: Loose, rattling with thick yellow pus. Stools: Foetid & offensive. Urine: With pus & mucus.
> Worse by	> Night, **New Moon and Full Moon,** open air, cold, noise, milk, sex, motion and mental exertion.
< Better by	< Warmth, summer, and passive motion.

TIPS FOR DIFFERENTIATING THE REMEDIES

a) Grouping the tissue salts

The three main groups

They are the **Calcium**, **Potassium**, and **Sodium** group. We can use the MENTAL TRAITS (from Homeopathy) to differentiate the tissue salts for treating constitutional disorders. Thus:

The **Calcium** trait usually puts a high value to stability and security. Hence, the person is usually 'nesting' and willingly plays a supportive role.

The **Potassium** trait is to be preoccupied with self-esteem issues like status and personal honour. Hence, the person will hold on to their views and react to blame.

And the **Sodium** person is always busy doing something, like tooling. And as a result people can find them to be emotionally unresponsive.

Differentiating the cleansing actions of the tissue salts

Intercellular fluids mainly contain **Sodium;** so the Sodium salts are helpful in cleansing the blood and lymphatic system.

The intracellular fluid mainly contains **Potassium;** so the Potassium salts are helpful in cleansing the nerves, glands and mucus membranes.

The deficiency of **mur** (chloride) salts give cough disorders;
the deficiency of **phosphate** salts give rise to weakness and
the deficiency of **sulf** (sulphate) salts give rise to an accumulation of toxins and have yellow discharges.

b) Tissue salts in Constitutional Disorders

Here we provide a one-line description for a quick differentiation of the tissue salt remedies:

Cal fluor

Loss of elasticity; calcification in joints and glands

Cal phos

Defective nutrition and weakness in muscles, bones and teeth

Cal sulf

Antiseptic for wounds that are discharging but not healing; useful for blood detox (removing pus)

Ferr phos

Poor circulation; lowered immunity; frequent infections and inflammations

Kali mur

Mucus membrane disorders; detox for lymphatic and glandular system

Kali phos

Nerve related troubles; auto-intoxication

Kali sulf

Skin disorders and hormonal disorders

Mag phos

Muscular cramps and nerve spasms; the biochemic aspirin

Nat mur

Excessive dryness or moisture; respiratory and digestive disorders; the biochemic antihistamine

Nat phos

Acidity; the biochemic antacid; stiffness in muscles and swellings in joints

Nat sulf

Toxaemia – high level of toxins in body fluids; excessive bile

Silicea

Weakness in connective tissue of mucus membrane, skin, hair and nails; constitutional weakness; offensive perspiration

c) *Treating Inflammations*

Consider the following order:

In the *first stage* when there is redness and temperature, use **Ferr phos**.

In the *second stage* when the temperature is less and there is congestion, use **Kali mur;** or if the discharge is fluent and watery, use **Nat mur**.

During the *third stage*, when expectoration has developed use **Kali sulf** (if expectoration is hard to expel), or **Cal sulf** (if it is easy to expel). These salts will increase the perspiration and complete the healing.

After the symptoms of inflammation have subsided, use **Cal phos** or **Sil** for a month to rebuild the immunity.

d) Treating an Abscess

While treating an abscess like a gumboil, treat the patient according to the particular stage in development of the ailment. Example:

In the beginning when the gums are red, hot and throbbing use **Ferr phos**.

When the redness has reduced and there is a swelling, but no pus use **Kali mur**.

When the pus forms slowly, or the boil remains blind for long, use **Sil** to ripen it.

After it is ripe use **Cal sulf** to clean it and close it.

However, if the suppurative process has become unhealthy and there are signs of some rotting shift to **Kali phos**.

Further, if the suppuration has affected the bone use **Cal fluor**.

e) Treating Pains

Back Pains: For pain due to weak elasticity of the tissue fibre and poor blood circulation, use **Cal fluor**;
for aching pain due weak bones or weakness in general, use **Cal phos**;
for pain due to acidity and digestive disorder, use **Cal phos** or **Nat phos**;
for pain due to nerve trouble, use **Kali phos**;
for pain due to weakness in connective tissue, use **Sil**.

Joint Pains: When pain is associated with excessive dryness or increased watery secretions, use **Nat mur**;
if it is due to weakness in the cartilage, use **Cal fluor** or **Sil**;
and when it is due to weakness in the bone, use **Cal phos**;

For pain *due to swelling,* use **Kali mur.**
For *shifting pains* as in rheumatism, use **Kali sulf.**
For pain due to *stiffness*, use **Nat phos**
For *muscular pain* that is sharp, cutting or cramping, use **Mag phos.**
And if the pain is *due to a boil* or an abscess, use **Sil**.

f) Treating Headaches

Use **Ferr phos** when the headache is accompanied by inflammation or acute disease. The headache is throbbing or congestive.

Use **Cal phos** when headache is accompanied by weakness or vertigo.

Use **Kali mur** when headache arises along with a stomach disorder and the tongue is coated white.

Use **Kali sulf** when headache arises in a heated room or in the evening.

Use **Kali phos** when the headache is nervous and one-sided or migraine.

Use **Mag phos** where the headache is accompanied by sharp pain

Use **Nat mur** when the headache is heavy and throbbing or caused by exposure to the Sun.

Use **Nat phos** when the headache is due to acidity; it is worse in the morning; and ache is dull and usually on the vertex, temporal or frontal region.

Use **Nat sulf** for bilious headaches (dull headache with nausea) that arise in the frontal or occipital region.

g) Tissue salts and Body Organs

Here the tissue salts are related to specific organs of the body.

Cal fluor

Elastic tissue of smooth muscles (of arteries, intestines, bladder, uterus and skin); tooth enamel, larynx and thyroid

Cal phos

Bones, muscles, tooth dentine, joint cartilage

Cal sulf

Liver, gall bladder, spleen, glands, mucus membranes, blood

Ferr phos

Blood, lungs and heart

Kali mur

Glands, throat, ear, mucus membrane

Kali phos

Brain, spleen, nerves, mucus membrane

Kali sulf

Skin, pancreas, liver, mucus membrane, endocrine

glands

Mag phos

Nerves in muscles, heart, colon, bladder, uterus

Nat mur

Kidney, liver, spleen, brain, blood, cartilage

Nat phos

Stomach, blood, lymphatic system, pancreas, intestines, kidney

Nat sulf

Liver, gallbladder, pancreas, colon

Silicea

Connective tissue of skin, hair and nails; cartilages, glands, nerve-sheath (cover)

h) Biochemic Ointments

The biochemic tissue-salts can be used as skin ointments. To prepare the ointment, crush one pill into a few drops of any non-medicated moisturizing lotion. Mix it without contact with metallic objects. Then apply the ointment on the skin just as you apply any lotion.

Cal fluor

Use it to soften hardened scars; to contract wrinkles on the face; to soften hardened tissues on the hands and feet; to tighten piles; to relieve cracked or chapped skin and to soften hard warts.

Cal phos

Use it to relieve pain from an old bone fracture. It will also relieve pimples in school girls.

Cal sulf

Use this salt where ulcer is purulent; when a boil is not healing; or there is fungal skin infection.

Ferr phos

Use it to relieve the bleeding in cuts and burses; in nose bleeding; and in bleeding haemorrhoids. You can also use it to sooth sunburnt skin.

Kali mur

Apply it on dry skin rashes where the scales are whitish or flour-like. It also helps in healing burns, blisters and soft warts.

Kali phos

Use it to relieve dull neuralgic pains and pain in shingles. It will also relieve muscular pain due to over exertion.

Kali sulf

Use it to relieve excessive sebaceous secretion as in Seborrhea Dermatitis. Apply it freely to skin that is itching, scaling or flaking

Mag phos

Use it to relieve muscular cramps and nervous spasms.

Nat mur

Use it to relieve nettle rash; and for eczema where there are blisters with a watery content.

Nat phos

Apply it where the skin is greasy or has blackheads. It also relieves skin irritation that is due to acidic perspiration.

Nat sulf

Use it for eczemas that are weeping; and where skin rashes have yellowish-green scabs or discharge.

Silicea

Use it to relieve scars and sensitive skin near the edges of nails. It will also relieve excessive and foul-smelling perspiration in the feet.

i) Tissue Salt indications from Facial Signs

Facial signs are also useful for diagnosing the biochemic cell salt deficiency. You can use it verify your diagnosis in constitutional disorders.

Cal fluor

There are folds and wrinkles below the eyes, and bluish-black colouring around the eyes. In older people the teeth enamel is worn out or the teeth have loose gums.

Cal phos

The skin is pale and waxy; and there is usually a 'stretched skin' appearance around the cheekbones. The lips are small and thin.

Cal sulf

There is dirty white colouring along the lower face or jaw; or brown spots appear on the face in old people.

Ferr phos

During an acute ailment the complexion is reddish; otherwise there is usually blue-black colouring under the eyes -- on the sides of the nose. The person has a 'hang-over' appearance and the face is pale.

Kali mur

Face skin is milky; there is thread-pulling saliva; the tongue is coated white; the eyes are glued together; and the glands are swollen.

Kali phos

The eyes are dull, they don't sparkle. The skin has ash-grey hue (colour); there is bad breath, bad body odour, and nervous sweating; and the tongue is brown and dry.

Kali sulf

There is brownish-yellow hue (colour) around the nose-mouth area; the eyelids are dark with yellow crusts; there are freckles; and there are skin scales like dandruff on a sticky base.

Mag phos

The cheeks are blushing (red); there is twitching of the eyebrows or the corners of the mouth.

Nat mur

The pores of the skin are large; the cheeks are

- e—

puffy; face is bloated; the lower eyelid has a bright gelatinous appearance. The rest of the skin is dry, itching, with dandruff.

Nat phos

Skin is greasy with many blackheads. The cheeks are hanging and there is a double chin. Metal jewellery gets discoloured due to acid skin.

Nat sulf

There are swollen bags below the eyes; the complexion has a shade of greenish-yellow.

Silicea

Face has a glossy-polish shine; the hairline has receded; there are dark circles and wrinkles around the eyes (crow's feet); the hair and nails are brittle (breaking).

THE PRESCRIPTION

Case taking

Begin a case by *writing down* the symptoms: Note the main complaint; observe the tongue; ask the nature of discharges; and use modalities (better by or worse by) or some peculiarity to differentiate the remedy.

Consider the remedy as indicated when any three guiding symptoms match of. Underline the symptoms on the basis of which you made your prescription.

Select the remedy on the basis of symptoms that stand out right now. Give greater importance to a strong symptom and allow it to dictate your pick.

Always start by treating the acute disorder. Consider only these symptoms. After the acute trouble has somewhat subsided, use the other symptoms to pick the chronic or constitutional remedy. Do not confuse the acute symptom picture with the chronic or constitutional disorder.

Repetitions

The normal prescription is to take 4 pills, 3 times a day. For children use 2 pills, and for infants use just one pill. Put the pills directly in the mouth and allow them to dissolve. Do not swallow.

Very often the symptoms of the case will be covered by two remedies. In such a case you should ALTERNATE the remedies. Allow time duration of a half-hour between the two remedies. Repeat each remedy 3 times in a day.

In acute cases, when the symptoms are intense and relief is urgently needed, repeat the dose every half-hour. After four repetitions there should at least be some signs of improvement. The patient should FEEL BETTER even if some of the symptoms of the disorder may continue or even get aggravated. After there is some relief, return to the schedule of 3 repetitions in a day.

However, if there is no noticeable improvement, consider changing the prescription. Take the case fresh and then decide the remedy once again on the basis of the symptoms that are standing out.

In acute disorders make the prescription for 2 to 7

days; and in chronic or constitutional disorders make the prescription for 2 to 6 months. Then once again record the symptoms and then reconsider your prescription. Continue it or change it according to the existing situation.

The pills should be taken at least a half hour after eating anything; and do not eat anything for at least 10 minutes after taking the pills.

Expect children to respond quickly to this therapy and old people to respond slowly.

In chronic cases do not permit the USE OF OTHER DRUGS along with this biochemic tissue salt treatment. If other medications are used, they will suppress the symptoms and disturb the natural working of the vital force. Then the body will be under dual stimulation. It will give confusing results.

However, in chronic cases it that is not always possible to have the patient discontinue taking drugs. So, tell the patient that after there is some improvement with these tissue salts they should reduce the dose of their prescribed drug, and if possible, to abandon the conventional treatment that merely suppresses the symptoms with drug therapy. It will not only reduce their dependency on drugs, but also avoid the harmful side-effects and after-effects that always arise from drug therapy.

Do 'side-effects' arise from using these tissue salts?

The active material in biochemic remedy is just a 'VIBRATION' that is carried in sugar. It is not a chemical drug. Therefore, if your prescription won't help the patient, it also won't do chemical or biological damage in the body. Further when you use the 6X potency, the dose will not significantly alter the symptom picture (which is something that happens when you use high potencies in homeopathy). Hence, it will not confuse another doctor who may have to subsequently take up your case.

What should you do when there is an aggravation of a symptom, like fever or a discharge, after taking or repeating the Biochemic remedy?

Don't get upset if there is an aggravation of symptoms during the treatment. The aggravation only indicates that the vital force of the body has been stimulated; and it has taken up the work of healing the body. Hence, it is a good sign. Then all you have to do is sit back and give some time for the healing to happen. When the vital force heals, the healing happens naturally. The results may not be as fast as in drug therapy, which that uses powerful drugs like antibiotics and steroids. However, since the healing happens as a natural process, it is much safer, surer, and it will also build your immunity to the disease.

Further, while treating chronic troubles, particularly the *skin ailments*, expect some symptoms will get aggravated during the healing process. The aggravation is a part of the healing, and if you use medicated applications to relieve these symptoms, you disturb the direction of the natural healing, which is 'inside out'. First the inner disorder has to be relieved and the symptoms must be allowed to come out to the surface. Then you may have to change the tissue salt according to the new symptom picture. In any case you must follow the case to complete it and not leave it half done.

In the same way when you treat *respiratory infections*, the acuteness of the symptoms is usually overcome in just a few days. However, thereafter the discharge will continue for some time. This happens because the body is using the opportunity to discharge the toxins that have accumulated in the cells. At such times the worst thing you can do is to suppress the symptoms with drugs. Instead, you should assist the healing process by correcting some of your diet and eating habits. The information for making these changes is given at the end of this book under the title *"Diet & Eating Habits"*.

Why there are no biochemic practitioners?

Many people, including homeopathic doctors, use these tissue salts in their everyday practice. However, people usually look for a 'lucrative profession' and the simplicity of this therapy does not allow that to happen. Hence, it is practiced by mothers, nurses and helpful neighbours. If you really want to help yourself, your family and friends, then this biochemic system will not disappoint you. The practice is intuitive; and your intuition will become very reliable as you continue to use it.

On Readymade Formulations

Today there are readymade formulations available in the market for common diseased conditions. They are prepared by *grouping all the tissue-salts that have a symptom that is COMMON to a disease.* The formulations usually consist of a combination of four tissue salts. They are very popular since they do not require careful case-taking. The commercial pharmacies also love them because they are big sellers! However, if effectiveness is the only criteria, the results got by using these 'wide spectrum formulations' can be disappointing.

The vibration of the tissue-salts gets diffused when they are given simultaneously as a combination. It could be that the effects of the tissue salts when taken together do not simply add up! Hence, we suggest that you do your homework to pick the correct remedy for your patient; if you pick two remedies, alternate them; and keep away from the readymade formulations that are marketed as 'remedies for classified diseases'.

Don't get upset when there is an aggravation of symptoms during the treatment. The aggravation only indicates that the vital force of the body has been stimulated; and it has taken up the work of healing the body...

When the vital force does the healing, the healing happens naturally. The results may not be as fast as in drug therapy, which uses powerful drugs like antibiotics and steroids. However, since the healing happens as a natural process, it is much safer, surer, and it will also build your immunity to diseases.

The worst thing you can do is to suppress the symptoms with drugs. Instead, you should assist the healing process by correcting some of your diet and eating habits.

REMEDIES FOR CLASSIFIED DISEASES

People always want a specific remedy for their specific ailment. To satisfy them to an extent, we have made a chart that shows the leading remedies for some common diseased conditions.

However, the tissue salts do not have a one to one correspondence with specific diseases. Hence, you should use the description given under the guiding symptoms to make a good prescription. You have to take the case in terms of the guiding symptoms, and not in terms of the clinical diseases.

Hence, the chart given below can only suggest the 'probable remedy'. You have to check the characteristic of the tissue-salt to see if it is 'the remedy' in your case.

Common Disorders	Leading Remedies
Abscess, boils with pus (painful)	Sil and then Calc sulf
Acidity, indigestion, heart burn, peptic ulcer	Nat phos
Anaemia	Ferr phos, Cal phos; Nat mur (for thin blood)
Arteriosclerosis (hardening of arteries)	Cal fluor
Asthma, humid	Nat sulf, Nat mur Chronic: Sil
Allergic rhinitis (cold, sneezing, headache)	Nat mur; also consider Kali mur, Kali sulf
Anxiety, tension	Kali phos; from grief: Nat mur
Bone and teeth tonic	Cal fluor, Cal phos, Sil
Bronchitis (wheezing), short breath; allergic	Ferr phos; Kali sulf; Kali mur

Common Disorders	Leading Remedies
Catarrh (stuffed up mucus membrane of nose and throat)	Congestion: Kali mur; dry or watery: Nat mur; chronic: Cal sulf, Kali sulf, Sil
Constipation	Dryness: Nat mur; with mucus Kali mur; with acidity: Nat phos; chronic: Sil
Corns	In feet: Sil; in palm: Nat mur
Colic – pain in abdomen	Mag phos; due to bad gas: Nat sulf
Cough	Kali mur, Kali sulf; intercurrent: Cal phos; chronic: Cal sulf
Cramps	Muscular: Mag phos; digestive: Cal phos; nervous: Kali phos

Common Disorders	Leading Remedies
Detox of:	*
Glands:	Cal phos, Kali mur
Blood:	Cal sulf
Nerves:	Kali phos
Skin:	Kali sulf
Water within organs:	Nat mur
Endocrine glands	Kali Sulf
Intercellular fluids:	Nat sulf, Kali mur
Diarrhoea	Nat phos, Nat sulf; Nat mur; chronic: Sil
Diabetes	Nat phos; Nat sulf
Dysentery	With blood: Ferr phos, Kali phos. With mucus: Kali mur, Kali sulf. With pus: Cal sulf
Depression	Nervous: Kali phos; from grief: Nat mur; from sadness: Nat sulf
Earache	Ferr phos, Kali mur, Kali

Common Disorders	Leading Remedies
	sulf
Eye infection	Cal sulf
Eczema	Dry & whitish: Kali mur; dry or watery: Nat mur; sticky & yellow: Kali sulf; wet: Nat sulf; chronic: Sil, Cal sulf
Epitasis, bleeding from the nose	Ferr phos, Cal phos
Fevers: Inflammation: To promote perspiration: Intermittent: Influenza (flu): Typhoid (high): Hay Fever	* Ferr phos Kali sulf Nat sulf; Nat mur Nat sulf; Kali mur Kali phos Nat mur, Nat sulf; Sil
Flatulence:	Nat sulf, Nat phos, Sil.

Common Disorders	Leading Remedies
Gas, belching:	Nat phos, Cal phos.
Hair loss due to dandruff:	Chronic: Sil; Kali sulf, Nat mur
Hives (Nettle rash)	Kali Sulf, Nat mur, Nat phos
Herpes Zoster (small painful water filled blisters along the nerve site):	Nat mur; second stage: Sil or Cal sulf; pain during: Kali phos
Hormonal disturbances	Kali sulf; Cal phos
Irritable, angry	Kali sulf, Nat mur
Ligament damage	Sil
Liver troubles	Jaundice: Nat sulf; congestion: Kali mur; abscess: Cal sulf
Mania (mental problems)	Kali phos; Nat mur

Common Disorders	Leading Remedies
Measles, chicken pox	Kali mur, Kali sulf
Mouth ulcers	Kali mur, Nat phos, Nat mur
Osteoarthritis	Spur: Cal flour; creaking due to dryness: Nat mur
Piles, haemorrhoids	Calc fluor
Pains	Nerve: Kali phos Cramping: Mag phos Swellings: Kali mur Bone/Cartilage: Cal Phos; Cal flour
Pimples, acne	Calc phos, Nat phos;
Rheumatism (muscular, fibrositis)	Nat phos, Nat sulf; with swelling: Kali mur; shifting pains: Kali sulf
Sinusitis	Congested: Kali mur; inflamed: Cal sulf;

Common Disorders	Leading Remedies
	chronic: Sil
Sleeplessness (Insomnia)	Nervous: Kali phos digestive: Nat phos, Nat Sulf
Stone in the kidney	To relieve pain: Mag phos; to dissolve stones: Sil & Cal phos
Suicidal disposition	Kali phos
Tonsillitis, pharyngitis, sore throat	Kali mur; chronic: Sil
Toothache	Kali phos
Ulcers	Sil, Cal Fluor, Cal sulf
Vertigo (giddiness)	Nervous: Kali phos; bilious: Nat sulf; weakness: Cal phos
Weakness, general debility, exhaustion	Kali phos, Cal phos; chronic: Sil

Common Disorders	Leading Remedies
Worms (in children)	Nat phos; then Cal phos
Warts	Soft: Nat sulf, Nat mur, Kali mur; hard: Sil, Cal fluor

A Review Request

Now that you have read the book, could I request you to grant me the favour by writing your review of the book on Amazon or Kindle Bookstore site?

It will do two things: It will tell others what they can realistically expect from reading this book; and it will tell us what you want or value so that we can, in future, produce the kind of books that will really benefit our readers. *Here are the steps:*

- Click Amazon.com or the Amazon site in your country.
- Sign into Amazon as you are prompted.
- Select an appropriate rating.
- Write a few honest words in the box that describe your impressions.
- Give your heading to the box.
- Click the 'submit' button

It's easy to do and I'll really appreciate it. Click on http://www.amazon.com/dp/B01FA6X4FG

Thanks,
Prashant

ABOUT THE AUTHOR

He was educated in Chemistry at Massachusetts Institute of Technology (BS), and University of California, (MS & PhC). He learnt Mantra Yoga from Shri Nyaya Sharma, a Master of Shiva-Tantra-Yoga; Homoeopathy from Post Graduate Homoeopathic Association, Bombay; he has healing hands and uses Pranic Healing. This book is an outcome of his personal experience of over 40 years.

The author conducts 'Correspondence Courses' through Darshana Centre, Vadodara, and 'Spiritual Awareness Workshops' in India, USA and UK. He speaks and writes clearly, in simple language, and from personal experience. His SITE on the Internet is at http://spiritual-living.in.

Other books by the author are: *The Crisis of Modern Humanity (1976); The Essence of Hindu Astrology (1987); The Practice of Mysticism (2009); The Art of Awakening the Soul (2011); Healing without Drugs (2014); Solving the Problems of Life (2015); and Restore your Health Naturally (2017).* The last 4 books are available from the Amazon Online Bookstore.

RESTORE YOUR HEALTH
NATURALLY

A time-tested way to heal yourself by simply changing your lifestyle and eating habits

ISBN-13: 978-1977555472; ISBN-10: 1977555470; The URL is https://www.amazon.in/dp/B075V5R1FJ

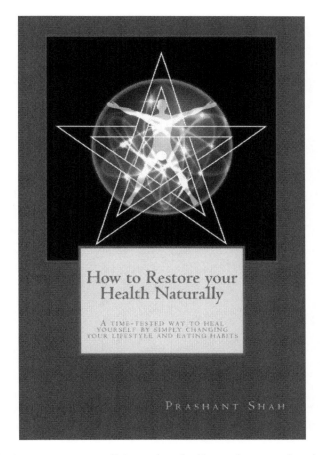

How to Restore your Health Naturally

A TIME-TESTED WAY TO HEAL YOURSELF BY SIMPLY CHANGING YOUR LIFESTYLE AND EATING HABITS

PRASHANT SHAH

Today we are conditioned to believe that our health depends on doctors, medicines, and the health care industry; whereas the truth is that our health really depends on our lifestyle, diet and emotions. When we understand this simple truth, we can learn to restore and maintain our health by our own efforts and, except in extreme cases, we will not need to consult doctors.

The method of natural healing is holistic and totally different from the specialised advice that you normally receive through the medical profession. It is simple; and to use it you do not need to know anatomy, physiology, pathology, toxicology or pharmacology. Further, the results got through this treatment are self-evident – so you don't have to depend on empirical proofs.

Your task is to simply strengthen the vital force of the body and help it in its effort to restore your health or keep you healthy.

Contents:

1. Foreword
2. Introduction
3. The medical profession focuses on relieving symptoms
4. What is so wrong with just relieving symptoms?
5. The holistic and analytic approaches to healing
6. Understanding disease in terms of toxaemia and the vital force
7. Aren't germs and bacteria the causes of

disease?

8. How to detoxify the body

9. Reduce the existing toxaemia

10. Avoid generating toxins

11. Correct your eating habits

12. On emotional causes

13. What causes the vital force to become weak?

14. The elimination crisis

15. If natural healing is so simple, why isn't everyone doing it?

16. Our message

From the book:

Diet and Eating Habits

Diet

Rule-1: Eat less, and take only easy-to-digest food. When you eat less food, you do not waste your energy on processing the excess food. When you can digest all the food you eat, you become more energetic and produce fewer toxins.

Rule-2: When food remains undigested in the body, it ferments. And that increases the toxin level in the body. Hence, value the food items *according to your ability to digest* and assimilate them, and <u>not</u> according to their nutrient content! Simply avoid eating food that is hard to digest or has toxic additives.

In specific:

- Avoid fried food, soybean preparations, sweets, chocolates, refined flour preparations and food containing preservatives.
- Avoid consuming food that is highly processed, highly sweetened or salted; or foods that carry health claims (don't encourage deceivers). Food is processed to increase its shelf life (not your life) and the processing makes it more indigestible in your body.
- Further, some foods are processed to make them tasty (deep-fried or addicting ingredients are added). It increases their consumption. However, that is better for the seller's business and not for your body.
- Avoid consuming 'concentrated' food-stuff. Don't be deceived by the label of extra nutrient value. They will be harder to digest. Instead, eat the food with lower nutritional value that comes with a lot of roughage and fibre. The fibre and

roughage make it easier for the body to digest and assimilate the food, and the waste products that are generated will also be easier to eliminate.

- Avoid consuming diet supplements and micronutrients unless you have a specific deficiency. Otherwise by taking them you serve the interests of the pharmaceutical companies, and not your interest. If you have a specific deficiency, take the supplement (preferably from a natural source) only until the deficiency is overcome. Do not continue to consume it thereafter. Otherwise it creates DEPENDENCIES and generates imbalance in the body. It is important to note that your deficiency arises due to weakened digestion and not due to insufficient intake. Once the digestion is restored, the body will, in most cases, overcome its deficiency naturally.
- If you suffer from allergies, consider milk and sugar as the culprits and give them up.

Eating habits

- The main purpose of eating is to feed the body.

Hence, do not combine other purposes, like parties and thrill with the act of eating.

- While eating, try to become conscious of what you eat, and how much you eat. When you maintain this discipline, the natural instinct of the body will awaken and allow you to sense the quality of the food you eat.
- Eat only two main meals in the day. Establish your meal time and adhere to it. Avoid eating between meals. Note: If you eat at odd times, you will not be hungry at the meal time! Further, if you don't get the 'hunger sensation' at meal time, don't eat. To eat at such times is injurious to health.
- Drinking water: You need at least nine glasses of water a day. Try to drink 'fresh stream' or mountain water; and avoid drinking tap water or recycled water. Further note: Drinking water is not the same thing as drinking beverages. You need fresh water and there is no substitute for it.
- The time factor: The morning time is naturally suited to the function of elimination. Hence, at this time avoid eating food, and drink of lot of water. The digestion is strongest around mid-

day. Hence, lunch should be your main meal. However, if it is not practical, you can make dinner your main meal, but take it early. Further, take rest after eating a big meal.

- The digestive fire becomes weak on overcast days and in the rainy season. Hence, eat less on such days and in the corresponding season.

Printed in Great Britain
by Amazon

75487897R00063